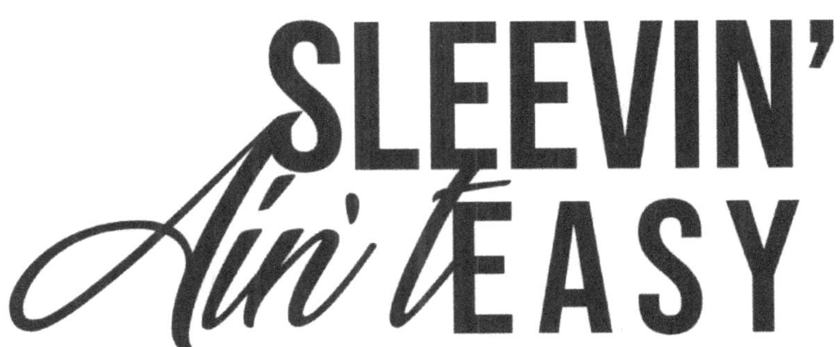

SLEEVIN' Ain't EASY

HOW SAYING 'I DO' TO WEIGHT LOSS SURGERY CHANGED MY LIFE

Tiberia Morris

DEDICATION

This book is dedicated to Mr. Jerry Wright and Kelvin Morris. Mr. Jerry was the very first man that called me pretty and told me I was "the pretty one" among my sisters. I had never heard that before. Being overweight for much of my life, I felt there was nothing pretty about me at all. One day Mr. Jerry called to speak to my daddy, and I happened to answer the phone. The voice on the other end said, "Hey, Pretty." I replied, "This is Tib!" Mr. Jerry then said, "I know who you are; the pretty one." That was the first time I had ever been called pretty by a man, or anyone for that matter. That one phone call to my daddy made an impact on my life that will never be erased. Mr. Jerry will forever be the voice that I hear when I don't feel pretty.

What can I say about my uncle Kelvin Morris other than he was my world? He was more than just my uncle, but a big brother (aka Big Bruh). He was the first to tell me the words: "Yes, you can." With tears in my eyes, I write this dedication to him because I would give anything to have him here with me now to see all that I have accomplished. His words keep me pushing forward, even today.

Thank you two men, for being the men that I needed to get to the woman I am today!

CONTENTS

INTRODUCTION: SAYING I DO TO ME

For years I've wanted to be skinny. I don't know why this was such an incessant desire. All I know is that I've never wanted something more desperately. Every ounce of my being wanted to be skinny from the moment I realized I was fat, and therefore a sore thumb among my peers and family. Being fat became my enemy very early on in my development. And before long, it became the guiding force in my life.

By the time I was old enough to attend school, I was always the fat girl in the group. That's even if I were a member of a group at all. Every single day of school was like entering a warzone. I battled an onslaught of name-calling hurled in my direction simply because I was fat. Not because I was a bad or unlikable person, but because my body mass index was higher than that of my classmates. Dodging ridicule day in and day out made attending school an exhausting task. It got so bad, overtime, that I often daydream about killing myself and leaving school (and this life) for good.

I had reached my heaviest adolescent weight when I was thirteen years old. Besides all of the other awkward and uncomfortable puberty changes I was experiencing, my body had ballooned to the size of an adult. I literally could fit my mother's clothing. But, what middle-schooler in her right mind wants to wear her mother's clothes? My large size was also the reason I was always chosen last to be on the volleyball or kickball team during PE. This social isolation from my peers was not only embarrassing, but it made me close off my true personality from the world. Therefore, when it came to boys and my growing interest in them, I never felt like I was pretty, worthy or skinny enough to gain the attention of any of my crushes.

To say that my grade school experience was humiliating is an understatement. I felt invisible for most of my school-aged years. It was like no one ever got to see or know the real Tiberia because they were immediately turned off by my weight. I constantly questioned myself. The cycle of self-deprecating questions was endless. Is this what my life is destined to be? Why am I like this? Am I capable of being loved? Do they really see me when they look at me? Am I ugly? Am I lovable? Am I always going to be fat?

These same questions traveled with me throughout high school and well into my adulthood when I had reached a staggering 401 pounds. But, by this point in my life I had become so good at being invisible, no one really knew how I felt about my weight. I had grown accustomed to going with the flow and smiling my way through life, even though under the surface a storm of uneasiness, doubt, fear and feelings of unworthiness always threatened to erupt beyond my calm and positive demeanor. I was able to keep the emotions at bay by eating my feelings away. The only problem with this remedy was that my food consumption never made the feelings disappear. The distraction of eating only provided a temporary redirection of my focus. And, more eating led to more weight gain, and climbing numbers on the scale led to more depression and questioning my value, which led to more eating. The cycle I was trapped in was endless and vicious.

I now know how common these kind of cycles are among fellow human beings. We all have felt inadequate in some area of our lives at one point or another. And instead of challenging these feelings with the truth of our potential and capabilities, we numb them with unhealthy alternatives. My drug of choice was food. For others it may be alcohol, controlled substances, people-pleasing, procrastination, avoidance or a plethora of other coping mechanisms. We choose temporary distractions because they give us a way out. More specifically an excuse not to feel what we feel. Society almost encourages us to exchange the act of confronting our feelings for anything that temporarily suppresses or numbs them. It's way more acceptable to be a zombie who lives in her head and is full of excuses than it is to get rid of the root of all detrimental thoughts and excuses: fear.

I can recall a memory when I was a child. It had snowed in Rome, Georgia and we lived at the top of a steep hill. My uncle wanted to take me outside to play in the snow and ride the toboggan down the hill. I didn't have any gloves, so he put 4 pairs of socks on my hands, and zipped me up in a big jacket with two scarves and we headed outside. I remember zooming down the hill and having so much fun with my uncle. But when we got to the foot of the hill, we couldn't go any further and had to turn around and head back up the hill.

At this time I wasn't really an obese child; I was slender with a little height. But trying to climb up that hill with all the layers of clothing I had on that were now heavy and wet from the snow seemed impossible. As we made our way up the hill—my uncle was a little further ahead of me—I remember stopping and yelling up to him. "Big Bruh" (this was my name for my uncle). "Big Bruh, I can't make it up the hill." He turned around and saw that I had stopped and yelled back, "Yes you can. Just keep going. You can make it." He coached me back up the hill with his reassuring words that day. Despite all the weight I was carrying from the bulky clothing I wore, I was still able to accomplish something I had initially deemed impossible.

My uncle's words came back to memory when I found adult Tiberia looking down at a scale that read 401 pounds. This was the heaviest I had ever been. My first instinct was to revert to my default setting of self-loathing, regret and emotional eating. But when I saw the shocking number, I sat in those feelings long enough to hear a voice from my past beckon me forward. You can make it. Just keep going. These same words led me to my decision to undergo weight loss surgery and years later write the book that you now read.

Writing this book has been an enormous challenge, to say the least. Unlike my first book, Say I Do To Greatness, I was required to really get completely transparent with my feelings as they relate to my weight. I had to say "I do" to Tiberia (and not just my purpose) and really be honest and courageous enough to shed the pounds I had longed to rid myself of for several decades. Herein, are the lessons that I learned after betting on myself for once and making my dreams come true.

As you read, prepare to go on a journey of finding your true voice in the midst of beating the battle of obesity.

I, like countless others, had to rediscover my voice by discovering the root of my emotional eating and obesity. I discuss my experiences of abuse, food addiction and lost and reclaimed self-esteem. This book will also address the stigmas associated with having weight loss surgery. I never imagined that undergoing a major surgery would be viewed as "the easy way out" by so many critics.

This book is my written testimony. I hope that you're able to find a piece of yourself in my story, whether your battling obesity, alcoholism, insecurities, self-doubt, fear, the urge to quit, depression, suicidal thoughts, molestation, mental wars, loneliness, or guilt. Today, you can make a decision to choose yourself and every single obstacle that has stopped you from living your best life. Your time is now.

CHAPTER 1: THE FATS OF LIFE

I learned about health, wellness and eating a balanced diet in elementary school. My teacher presented the class with a vibrantly colored pyramid that depicted the hierarchy of the five food groups. Fruits and vegetables were shown on the first layer. A level above that were grains and starches, followed by the dairy category. Above the milk and cheeses were the fats and oils. And at the very top were the sugary and salty processed foods, known as the snack and junk food category. I recall the layers and my teacher telling the class that we should eat more fruits and vegetables than we did snacks. We discussed specific serving sizes, but in my house, this type of variety and portion control was none existent.

I grew up in a southern household where the food was delicious and laden with all the fats, oils, sugars and starches that should have been consumed in moderation, according to my nutrition pyramids from school. But, there was nothing moderate about the heaping serving size of food given to me as a child. Second helpings were a normal occurrence at my dinner table. My family also practiced the eat-before-you-drink rule. Basically, I was reprimanded for trying to take a sip of my juice or soda before eating all the food on my plate. And since I really wanted to enjoy my beverage during dinner, I would rush my eating so that I could quench my thirst. I now know that rushing one's eating doesn't give the stomach's "I'm Full" sensor time to register in the brain, which inevitably leads to overeating. Learning to override these sensors as a child so that I could drink my beverage led to the makings of a 400-pound woman who ate up to four full helpings of food before feeling satisfied.

At my grandmother's house I learned that food could be the ultimate comfort and companion. Grandmothers just have a way of making their homemade cuisine feel like a warm hug. And my grandmother was not shy about making sure that we ate our fill of food. "Go on a get some more food, Tib" were comforting words in my grandmother's house. She would say this anytime she felt that I was still hungry or wanted another serving of her delicious food. My grandmother took pride in feeding her grandchildren and I developed a yearning to always feel the comfort I felt when eating her food. My grandmother's harmless beckoning to help myself to more food became my safe place, especially as I endured unmentioned traumas during those early years. Food became my comfort zone, happy place, boredom blocker, friend, lover, dependent and peace of mind. In fact, I felt safe when I was eating.

Looking back on those times, I realize that food became my everything. I was obsessed with food because getting my fill of food was the only way I felt loved. I really thought that the food I consumed, loved me in return. But as the calories increased and the pounds packed on, I realized that my one friend began to betray our relationship by making me miserable in my own skin. This betrayal nearly ruined my life and destroyed my purpose before it even had a chance to grow and blossom.

Being the only overweight child in my family created a world of tumultuous internal emotions that I would never want any child to ever experience. Normal shopping trips to purchase school clothes became a dreadful occurrence for me. When I was ten, I remember feeling like the late Michael E. Duncan in the movie, Green Mile. I was so afraid that every time I walked into a department store, I would have to leave empty handed because I was too big to fit any of the clothing. I desperately wanted to be small like my sisters and wear regular sizes. I remember going to a popular clothing store called Amy's with my mom and sister and being mortified that I could not fit anything in the store. Instead of wearing the stylish fashions found in that store, I had to wear clothes with big ugly flowers on them and stretch pants. I hated stretch pants! But I had to wear them throughout my entire teenage and young adult life.

My fragile self-esteem took a blow with every shopping trip. I began to equate my difficulty for finding clothes that fit me with being ugly and unattractive. I constantly questioned myself. Why am I so fat? How did I get this fat? Why couldn't I just stop eating? Why couldn't I lose the weight? Why did I have to be the FAT one? Every night I would close my eyes and pray that I would wake up in a new, smaller body. My prayer was never answered.

Going to high school was said to be an emergence into one's "Glory Days". This was the time when adolescence became young adults and really began to figure out who they were and what they wanted to pursue in life. To say that my high school experience was less than glorious is an understatement. Being teased and made fun of because I was fat became my normal reality. This mental and emotional abuse at the hands of my peers was daunting to say the least. I felt under constant attack because of obesity. In fact, I later viewed obesity as my actual abuser, because this state of being was my greatest foe.

When I was a senior in high school, I wanted nothing more than to be chosen for a senior superlative. I at least thought I was smart enough to get Most Likely To Succeed, but I quickly realized that these coveted titles were only given to students who were popular and thin. When it was time for senior prom, I had worked up the nerve to write a letter to the finest guy in my school, asking him to prom. He was my friend, so I thought I had a chance. Instead of writing a response to my letter, Mr. Popular told me that he had decided not to go to prom. I was puzzled. How could one of the most popular and best looking guys at our school not go to senior prom? But, I didn't question his response.

By this time, I weighed about 380 pounds, so finding a prom dress was very difficult. But luckily, my mom was an excellent seamstress. I found a really pretty pattern at the local sewing store, and purchased some fabric and let my mom work her magic. She was so excited to sew my first prom dress. I shared in her excitement, but was still anxious about not having a date. At the time, I didn't have a driver's license, so I knew that not having a date who drove would probably result in me forfeiting my senior prom experience. But, at the eleventh hour, I asked my younger cousin Qiana if should would attend prom with me if I talked my uncle into letting us borrow his car. She agreed and my uncle loaned us his car, so Operation: Senior Prom Night was underway.

I had made dinner reservations at Red Lobster before prom started. When I arrived, I was shocked by who I saw sitting at a close by table. That's right, my friend and Mr. Popular was decked out in his prom attire sitting with his date! I was devastated. Instead of telling me the truth that he had decided to take someone else to the prom, he thought it was okay to blatantly lie to me. And I really thought he was my friend. To make matters worse and more awkward, he spent the entire time at Red Lobster talking to me as if he did not even have a date. The thoughts that ran through my mind concerning him were not nice or kind in any shape or form. But, I was determined not to let this little faux pas ruin my senior prom, and my friends and cousin made sure of that. I had a blast at prom, but the lingering thought in the back of my mind was why had I really been rejected by a guy I really liked?

CHAPTER 2: SILENT CRIES

Being constantly teased about my weight and outward appearance as a teenager, eventually created a very distinct inner and outer version of Tiberia as an adult. On the outside, I smiled and appeared to be confident. I always had an encouraging word for others, and people from all walks of life genuinely enjoyed my company. But on the inside, I was an emotional wreck. My thoughts attacked my mental wellbeing on a daily basis. I constantly questioned my value, worth and reason for letting myself get to such a place where I hated the way I looked externally. These mental battles were so overwhelming and futile to my self-esteem that they often led me right back into the hands of my abuser: food.

Eating was a shelter and safe haven for me, even though I knew that constantly eating was the reason why I packed on the pounds and hated more and more the skin I was in. But in those moments of silent soul cries, I really saw no other alternative. Suicidal thoughts were a regular occurrence in my psyche. Sometimes it just seemed like it would be easier to just leave this physical world instead of straddling the fence between the character I played on the outside and the ugliness I endured on the inside. And where were all those people that I had encouraged when I needed to have my encouragement cup filled?

Food was my addiction. I finally admitted this truth after I became an observer of my habits. Whenever I felt sad, happy, in control or out of control, I ate. It really didn't matter what emotion I felt, they all triggered my desire to eat. And not just eat for nourishment, but binge eat until I no longer knew what it felt like to be full. I can remember one particular time when I had eaten a full course meal, but when I finished, it felt like I literally had not eaten at all. So I kept eating until I finally felt the comfort of fullness. However, by this time, I was completely sick to my stomach.

This cycle of binge eating and beating myself up emotionally finally came to a head one day while I was in church. I was sitting in the sanctuary during a prayer of declarations that the pastor was saying over the congregation. We were approaching a New Year, so he began each of his statements with "This year you will...". When he said this year you will lose the weight, his proclamation shook me to my core. It's as if God himself was talking directly to my spirit. I repeated this word to myself saying, "Tiberia, this year you will lose the weight." And in that moment, I accepted this affirmation as the undeniable truth.

Before this experience in church, I had succumbed to a life of settling into the fact that I was morbidly obese. I did not see any other way of existing in the world. I had dieted and tried making healthier eating choices in the past, but they all landed me back into a cycle of food addiction and binge eating. I saw no way out of this cycle. But, after saying those words to myself and believing them, I knew I had been given access to an exit strategy that would release me from both my physical and emotional bondage once and for all.

CHAPTER 3: NIGHTMARE ON LION KING STREET

In 2015, the Broadway musical, The Lion King came to Atlanta. I had always wanted to see the show so I scoured the Internet for tickets. Unfortunately, my search came up empty handed. Tickets for the Fox Theater were completely sold out. I was devastated. I told my then husband, about there being no available tickets, and he came up with the plan for us to travel to a nearby state to see the show. So we located tickets in Philadelphia and the plan to see The Lion King was back on.

I had never been to Philadelphia, so the excitement of touring a new city with my husband was overflowing. Plus, Philadelphia was the capital of cheesesteaks, so I had already planned out how I would partake freely of the tasty offerings available in this food haven.

We purchased our tickets to the show, booked a hotel room and purchased outfits with the same color scheme to wear the night of the show. But, when we arrived in Philly, a few weeks later, there was an issue with our hotel room. Determined to maintain my excitement, I told my husband that I would speak with the front desk clerk about the pricing issue. Once our conversation was completed, everything was rectified, and Operation Lion King in Philadelphia was on in full effect.

Day Two in Philadelphia was all about sightseeing. Our first stop was the "Rocky Steps" in front of the Philadelphia Museum of Art. There were only 72 stairs to climb, but at my size, it seemed like 50 million! Let's just say, I didn't make it all the way to the top. With every step I took, I was out of breath. And not to mention, my back was hurting and the excruciating pain in my knees was almost unbearable. But, I didn't want to ruin the trip with all my ailments and complaints, so I did what I knew best; I quit. I stopped part way up the steps, and when I say part way, I had probably climbed about 20 steps successfully. But standing 5 feet 3 inches at 385 pounds in the 100-degree Philadelphia heat, quitting and finding the nearest park bench was the only thing on my mind. But my journey didn't stop there. My husband wanted to walk to the museum. I obliged his request, because I too wanted to see as much of Philadelphia as I could. It was just that my body had other plans.

I truly pushed myself physically that day in Philadelphia. As we walked down the crowded and busy streets, my feet were screaming and pleading for me to rest them with every step. But, I forged on in silent pain. I was already uncomfortable because of the resistance my body was experiencing as a result of physical activity, but to make matters worse, the stares from onlookers were incessant. Complete strangers ogled me as if I were an unknown creature from a planet other than earth. I tried my best, however, to ignore the disdain, disgust or pity I perceived in their faces and enjoy my vacation with my husband.

We walked all over the museum, took pictures and enjoyed the scenery of a new location together. When it was time for us to leave, sheer dread entered my mind as I thought about the great distance we had to walk back to Silver Bullet. That was the name we had given our four-door Honda Civic. I braced myself for more pain and took the long journey back to our car. I was never so happy to see our vehicle than on that day in Philly. My body was definitely put to the strain test, and I was paying for it tremendously. But, all that was just the prequel to what was to come.

It was Day Three in Philadelphia, and finally the long awaited time to see The Lion King had come. My husband and I woke up so excited. We had been planning for this day for weeks. Our matching outfits proved this. I couldn't be any happier that morning. For one, I was married to an awesome man, and two I was getting to experience new surroundings and see a performance I had always dreamed of seeing. But little did I know, my excitement would soon be sullied with one of the greatest tasks that I would ever have to face in my life.

As I put the finishing touches on my outward appearance, I looked in the mirror and told myself I was beautiful. Even if I only partially believed it, I still shared those pleasantries with myself that day.

When Greg and I got in the car, we had huge grins on our faces. We left our hotel early enough to get a good parking space, but to our surprise, show guests were given valet parking services. That was awesome because it meant that I didn't have to worry about walking too far of a distance. And considering my experience the day before, being let out at the entrance of the theater was a definite plus.

When I stepped out of the car, the strap on my cute and comfy pair of black sandals popped. Looking back on this, I consider this snafu a foreshadowing of what was to come. My husband hadn't noticed my wardrobe malfunction, so I tried my best to walk as normally as possible. No broken sandal strap was going to steal my joy.

As we made our way inside the theater, there was a long queue for the elevator. My husband and I didn't want to risk missing the actual curtain opening, so we did the unthinkable (lol) and decided to take the stairs.

At first glance, the stairs at the theater didn't look as daunting as the Rocky Steps. But after I had cleared the first flight, my knees began to hurt, my back began to spasm, my body heated up and I felt perspiration coating my skin. I kept going, however, and made it to the last step. I had won the battle.

Once we reached the section where our seats were situated, I entered into a war that nightmares of obese men and women are made of. I stared at the size of the seats in our row, and immediately knew that I was in for a long night. Sheer embarrassment gripped my heart and spread across my face as I accepted my fate. I wished in that moment that my husband and I could have just turned around and left, or better yet, had purchased tickets in the sections that were filled with regular chairs. But none of these scenarios were happening, so I faced the music of my Nightmare on Lion King Street.

As I walked to my seat, I felt like I was taking the strides that the late actor Michael Duncan took in the movie The Green Mile. When Greg and I sat down, he tried to better position himself to get comfortable; he was overweight too. But since I was much heavier than he, I just tried to get myself in a bearable position in which I could remain for the next three or four hours. As I maneuvered in the cramped seat, I prayed that no one else would have to sit next to me. But, just as quickly as my prayer made it to God's ears, there was a skinny man standing at about 6 feet 4 inches walking down the aisle to take his seat next to me. Needless to say, the gentleman was very friendly and chatted with me and my husband before the curtain opened. But, all I could really think about was: what is this man really thinking about me? Is my fat making him uncomfortable? Because it sure as hell is making me uncomfortable.

That evening in a dark theater, I met the reality of just how big I had gotten. If I had not known the truth before then, there was no denying that I had allowed myself to balloon to a size that had now stolen the joy out of my Lion King experience. The opening act came and ended and I was semi-comfortable, minus the embarrassment that made me want to forfeit seeing the rest of the performance. But, like the saying goes, the show must go on. And that it did all the way to the first intermission.

By this time, my knees had began to hurt. But when the other show attendees got up to stretch their legs or use the restroom, I stayed glued to my seat. The embarrassment of my obesity and inability to properly make my body fit comfortably in my chair was paralyzing. So, I just grunted through the pain and sat there.

Before Act Two began, I turned to my husband with a sincere look on my face and told him I had reached my breaking point. I could no longer live like this. Up until that moment, I had not realized the large space my size occupied. In fact, I later learned that lots of people who are obese deal with this same issue. When we look at ourselves in the mirror, we just see us. But, the truth of our size is shockingly revealed to us in photos. The pictures that I saw of myself from that night were alarming. I had no real clue about how big I truly was. Facing this revelation in such a public venue is probably one of the most humiliating moments of my life, if I'm honest.

Before the third and fourth acts began, I forced myself to get up and stretch. My body was in so much pain, and my sides and back were scraped and bruised from the stuffing and squeezing they had to undergo as I shifted back and forth in my seat. When I stood up I felt like biscuits that had just received their freedom papers from the can when it pops open from all the built up pressure.

Seeing the Broadway performance of The Lion King was supposed to be one of the happiest moments of my life. I was supposed to share a wonderful outing with my husband. Instead, when the curtain rose for the final act, I was relieved that I wouldn't have to be subjected to the tight squeeze on my chair for much longer. My discomfort, embarrassment and pain had overshadowed my entire evening. In fact, my seating arrangement began to spotlight an even bigger issue in my life.

I had grown so comfortable with being obese that the tight chair made me realize just how uncomfortable obesity truly was. For years, I had tried to lose weight with dieting, meal replacement shakes and signing up with companies like Weight Watchers and Jenny Craig. I even had gone as far as getting a prescription for diet pills, which worked for a moment. I had lost a significant amount of weight and even maintained it. But once I started dating my now ex-husband, I re-entered a space of complacency which led to increased weight gain. And from that point, I gave in to the idea that being morbidly overweight was my destiny. But after that night in Philadelphia, I was fed up. I could not wait any longer to lose the weight that had consumed my entire life.

On the ride back to our hotel room after the show, I told my husband that I was going to start researching weight loss surgery. And this time when I found the right physician, I was going to follow through with the procedure. In the past, I had attended seminars and hadn't completed the journey to receive bariatric surgery. But the dark cloud my weight had casted over what could have been a magical night was my tipping point. I was all in. There was no turning back. Weight loss surgery was the answer to my question and a risk I was finally willing to take.

CHAPTER 4: SLEEVIN' AND LEAVING

September 03, 2015

Today is the big day! I am about to change my whole life and be on the "Losers" bench with thousands of women and men that have made the decision to have the gastric sleeve operation. I am so scared; I hope I am not in too much pain. I really feel like a weight is about to be lifted off of me. In fact, more than 100 pounds will soon be gone forever from my life. I have such a peace about this decision. I know it won't be easy and the challenge is going to be great, but I think I am finally going to meet the girl I have always longed to meet.

After much research and prayer, I decided to undergo gastric sleeve surgery on September 3, 2015. In the bariatric and weight loss surgery community, this technique is called sleevin' for short. There are numerous weight loss surgeries available to those who need them. The one I chose to help save my life was a sleeve gastrectomy. I learned that this type of surgery is a very popular choice for helping win the battle over obesity. This option didn't run the risk of long-term complications or require maintenance. Sleevin' was also said to have seven other benefits besides weight loss.

The gastric sleeve was said to:

- Reduce hunger
- Have a shorter operation time compared to the gastric bypass
- Not reroute intestines
- Cause no dumping syndrome
- Require no adjustments like the Lap-Band may need if the band slips or moves.
- Eliminate the need for a foreign object left in the body, like a Lap-Band.
- Help weight loss occur over a period of 18 months

Before I move on with my personal weight loss surgery experiences, I want to take the time to provide some additional information about the different types of bariatric surgeries available. This section is just an overview, and should not be taken as medical advice. This is just a collection of my findings and answers to frequently asked questions. Please contact a professional healthcare provider who specializes in bariatric surgery if you are interested in receiving help for obesity.

Understanding Obesity Surgery: Here's What's Involved

Obesity surgery is also known as weight loss surgery. A more technical term would be bariatric surgery. There are actually several types of bariatric surgeries. If you're looking to lose weight and reverse obesity then surgery may be an option.

Who is Obesity Surgery For?

Obesity surgery is often prescribed for individuals whose health is at extreme risk. For example, if blood pressure or cholesterol is at dangerous levels a doctor may believe surgery is the best option. However, obesity surgery isn't an easy fix. People who undergo obesity surgery have to be committed to lifestyle changes. The surgery demands it. And recovery can take quite a while. Weight loss surgery is only recommended if a person is motivated to lose weight and dedicated to the process.

Other Types Of Obesity Surgery

The most common type of obesity surgery may be Gastric Bypass, however, there are a total of seven types of weight loss surgeries. With the gastric bypass procedure the surgeon staples closed a large portion of your stomach. The remaining stomach size holds about an ounce of food. It's about the size of a walnut. Your intestine is then relocated to connect to this smaller stomach. During this surgery patients undergo general anesthesia.

Some physicians perform the surgery with a laparoscope. A small tool, tube shaped with a camera at the end. The surgeon then only has to make a small incision in your abdomen and you have a shorter hospital stay.

After the surgery you won't be able to eat for a few days. After that patients are on a liquid diet for several weeks. You'll gradually graduate to pureed foods and then to solid foods. This specialty diet lasts approximately three months. After that, you'll only be able to eat very small amounts of food. You'll also have to eat them very slowly. Too much too fast and you'll vomit. It can be quite painful.

Most patients lose fifty to sixty percent of their weight in the first two years. So the surgery works. However, you want to make sure you're willing to live with the new lifestyle and recovery time required.

The Lap Band

The Lap Band surgery is another type of weight loss surgery. With this surgery, doctors place a band around the top of your stomach. It has the same effect of reducing your stomach size. However, unlike a Gastric Bypass, the surgery doesn't require your intestines to be relocated. The Lap Band instead restricts the flow of food from the top of your stomach to the bottom of your stomach. This gives you a sense of fullness so you don't overeat.

The Lap Band is also adjustable and doctors will re-evaluate your Lap Band approximately four to six weeks after surgery. With both types of surgeries there is a risk of death. There are other potential side effects and risks with obesity surgery. There are also significant recovery periods for both surgeries. If you believe you're a candidate for weight loss surgery talk with your doctor about all of the risks and requirements for the surgery. It's a weight loss solution that has changed many lives for the better. However, it doesn't come without risks.

Gastric Balloon

The Intragastric balloon known as gastric balloon allows you to temporarily feel full sooner while eating (balloon removed after 6 months). The gastric balloon is inserted orally through your esophagus and placed directly into your stomach during a quick, non-surgical procedure. The 20-minute procedure is completed while you are mildly sedated. Most patients go home to start their weight loss journey on the same day. After the first six months of the weight loss program the stomach balloon is carefully removed and the aftercare program continues. Since the weight loss balloon is inserted through your throat and into your stomach there is no need for any incisions, stitches or scars.

Duodenal Switch

The Duodenal Switch surgery is a variation of another procedure, called biliopancreatic diversion. But duodenal switch leaves a larger portion of the stomach intact, including the pyloric valve, which regulates the release of stomach contents into the small intestine.

As the name suggests, the duodenal switch also keeps a small part of the duodenum in the digestive system. The duodenum is the first part of the small intestine.

It is located between the stomach and the jejunum, or the middle part of the small intestine. With the duodenal switch, you consume less food than normally, but it is still more than with other weight loss surgeries. Even this amount of food cannot be digested as normal, so a large amount of food passes through the shortened intestines undigested. The procedure can also be performed laparoscopically, meaning that your surgeon makes small incisions as opposed to one large incision. He or she inserts a viewing tube with a small camera (laparoscope) and other tiny insert instruments into these small incision.

vBloc Therapy

Delivered via a pacemaker-like neuroregulator device, vBloc Therapy blocks hunger signals between the brain and stomach, which can make you feel fuller longer and reduce the amount of food you want to eat. The device is placed just under the skin. The leads are placed on the trunk of the vagus nerve. Because the leads are placed laparoscopically, there is limited scarring and recovery time compared to traditional bariatric surgeries. Better yet, many patients are able to have the procedure done on an outpatient basis to perform duodenal switch.

AspireAssist

The AspireAssist works by reducing the calories absorbed by the body, while helping patients make gradual, healthy changes to your lifestyle. After eating, food travels to the stomach immediately, where it is temporarily stored and the digestion process begins. Over the first hour after a meal, the stomach begins breaking down the food, and then passes the food on to the intestines, where calories are absorbed. The AspireAssist allows patients to remove about 30% of the food from the stomach before the calories are absorbed into the body, causing weight loss. You'll also need to chew carefully and eat mindfully, which helps give time for the fullness signals from your stomach to reach your brain.

A thin tube will be placed in your stomach that connects the inside of your stomach directly to a discreet button on the outside of your abdomen. After each meal, the device enables you to empty, or "aspirate", up to 30% of your meal into the toilet through this tube by connecting a small, handheld device to the button. The device is about the size of a smartphone, and stores away in a small case afterwards. The aspiration process is performed about 20 to 30 minutes after the entire meal is consumed and takes 5 to 10 minutes to complete. The process is performed in the privacy of the restroom, and the food is drained directly into the toilet. Because aspiration only removes a third of the food, the body still receives the calories it needs to function.

The next set of research is specific to gastric sleeve surgery, and the questions that I needed answered before I made a decision.

How fat or obese do you have to be to have the gastric sleeve?

Before you can receive gastric sleeve surgery, the National Institute of Health requires you to be more than 100 pounds overweight as a man and more than 80 pounds overweight as a woman. This procedure combines a high weight-loss success rate with little side effects.

Potential gastric sleeve complications and side effects include:

- Staple line leaks
- Bleeding
- Stenosis/strictures
- Digestion issues
- Sagging skin from rapid weight loss
- Divorce
- Loss of friendships

Most people won't choose this option because they think or have been led to believe that death would be their ultimate fate if they go through with it. This is so far from the truth, in fact the 30-day mortality rate for sleeve gastrectomy was 0.08 percent, while the rate for gastric bypass was 0.14 percent and 0.03 percent for gastric banding. These mortality and complication rates are lower than those typically associated with gallbladder or hip replacement surgery.

After conducting several months of research, I decided to go with the gastric sleeve. This one decision was the beginning of an avalanche of changes that would take place in my life. Some of the transitions were welcomed and others completely blindsided me. All in all, I want to help dispel the myth that opting for weight loss surgery is the easy or lazy way out of the battle against obesity. This notion could not be further away from the truth. In fact, it's quite common that those who undergo bariatric surgery have to work ten times harder than those who lose weight naturally.

There was nothing easy about planning to have weight loss surgery for four years and then backing out right before the operation stage. There is nothing easy about being gripped with the fear that you may not wake up after the anesthesia wears off. There was nothing lazy or easy about having to battle the emotional and mental warzone that arose within me at the mere thought of finally getting to live as the person I always knew I was.

At 37 years old, I contemplated with the idea of going under the knife. I had even convinced myself that if God wanted me to have a smaller stomach, he would have given it to me. I can laugh at this statement now, but trust me the fear I had when declaring it was no punch line.

I remember talking to my friend Nyasia one day. I was venting about how I hated myself, and the way I looked and felt. But I told her that I was so afraid of not waking up from anesthesia that I felt stuck. In a very matter-of-fact tone, she told me that I needed to do what I needed to do in order to improve the health, wellbeing and longevity of my life. She even added that there was no way I would die on the operating table because I had too much left to accomplish here on earth. The words she spoke to me on that occasion, gave me the strength to move forward with my decision to have gastric sleeve surgery.

The weeks preceding my surgery were filled with lectures, classes and evaluations that I had to undergo. There were nutrition classes, lectures that discussed the do's and don'ts of life after surgery and even psychological evaluations. My doctor needed insight into whether or not I was capable mentally and emotionally handling gastric sleeve surgery and recovery. Dealing with the emotional effects of surgery on bariatric patients was one thing that was rarely discussed. In fact, as a sleevivor, I found it extremely difficult to get a handle on my emotions, especially as a recovering emotional eater.

Emotional eating is what had led to my morbid obesity. I ate in order to stuff my feelings. And there was always a side of me that knew that this type of eating was not normal and problematic, but I still force-fed myself. Obesity was my prison, and I had sentenced myself to a constant cycle of keeping my stomach full in order to avoid hidden emotions that were starving for attention. When I made the decision to have weight loss surgery, I had to be certain that I was willing to give up the way I saw food. My skewed perception of eating had to be remedied if I was to truly experience a life transformation.

My surgeon's name was Dr. Michael Williams. I consider him my Moses. He brought me out of the land of obese Egypt and into my promised land that flowed with health, wealth, milk and honey. In this new territory, I had higher self-esteem, greater confidence and a boldness that no one could rob me of. He led me through the final hours of my wilderness experience, and on September 3, 2015, I was reborn.

From the moment I stepped foot inside the hospital, I had this overwhelming sense of freedom. I felt like a prisoner having her last walk through the correctional facility before being released. I was nervous, and a little scared, but every cell in my being knew that I was making the right decision in order to save my life. The trajectory of my path would never be the same. In fact, the changes that were destined to occur were already taking place.

On the day of my surgery, I was alone. The support that I thought I had from my then husband was non-existent on one of the most important days of my life. Things were dramatically transitioning in my marriage, and it seemed like my decision to unload years of weight was the catalyst of this shift.

For those considering weight loss surgery, it may be both the best and most challenging decision you'll ever make. If you think not eating and drinking is hard, you can only imagine having to drink 64 ounces of water each day. This was one of my biggest struggles. Everything else came pretty easy for the most part.

Getting over my food addiction was just half the battle. I went from engaging in unmonitored eating habits and a no exercise regimen to contemplating the price of my freedom. As I previously mentioned, obesity was my jail so I had to think about what I was willing to pay for my freedom. What would it truly cost me? What would I have to give up? Would I really be willing to sacrifice what was necessary to help solidify my success? Was I willing to give up my skewed perception of food, and trade my large portions into smaller more suitable ones? Was I willing to give up my old way of living for a new lifestyle that I had only dreamt about? These questions swam around in my head.

When I finally made the decision to go all in with a new way of living, I was hit with a double whammy—two divorces. Not only did I have to divorce my old way of thinking about and knowing Tiberia Sheree Morris, I had to divorce food. Well not food altogether, but I had to divorce my unhealthy relationship with food. More specifically, I had to sever the stronghold that comfort food had over my life. I had to break up with fast food and sodas. Sodas were tough to give up, but the hardest relationship to lose was my undying devotion to bread. Bread was literally one of my most favorite things to eat. But, I had to let it go to save my life. Little did I know, however, divorcing my favorite foods registered low on the emotional Richter scale compared to the big tie that was soon to be dismantled.

September 21, 2015

I am starting to regret my decision. Why? Because every time I look in the mirror I still see 385 pounds. I can't tell that any weight is falling off and I want to eat regular food so badly. God, I hate what I've done to my body, and now I have to fight like hell to undo the damage I caused. I am at home feeling unwanted by the very person that said 'til death do us part. He isn't really here for me, at least not like I thought he would be. He didn't even think enough to take off his job to even be with me at the hospital or even after I came home. I know he is working to keep the money rolling in, but I would have thought he would have at least been with me as they rolled me into the operating room. This still hurts me to my core. I guess that's why I am writing about it now because I am still emotionally affected by this.

At this point though, I can't give up and I can't undo what I have done. I have to just trust the process of this surgery and don't rush it. Sigh. Maybe after I have lost some weight, he will want to be with me sexually. Hell, I ain't had none in months; almost seven months. That is half the time of our one year marriage. I am trying to remain positive and keep fighting until I lose all the weight I desire to lose.

The Leaving

December 14, 2014 was the best day of my life. It was the day I married my best friend, or at least that is what I thought. But just six months after my surgery, my whole world turned upside down. Writing this chapter brings so many emotions to the surface. But I desire to share my truth, because I share a similar truth with countless others who have had weight loss surgery.

A few months after my surgery, my husband of one year and three months decided not to return home. After many days of asking what was wrong, and inquiring if he was coming home, I began to question my entire decision of pursuing and even having weight loss surgery. The night before April Fool's Day in 2016, my husband returned home to discuss why he hadn't been home. Nothing could have prepared me for the words I heard that night. He came in, sat on the bed and began his explanation for disappearing. He told me that he had done a lot of things wrong in his life, and that he had made many mistakes. He followed this line with a whole bunch of other words that went in one ear and out the other. Nothing he was saying made any sense or properly explained why he had disappeared. He then hit me with news that nearly knocked the wind out of me.

My spouse of eighteen months told me that our marriage was not legitimate. He followed this verbal sucker punch with the news that his previous divorce was not finalized and he was still legally married to his first wife. I was so emotionally spent and vulnerable by this development that I just believed his story. My only follow-up question was, "Do you want to get remarried?" He said, "I need to get MY life together." I was speechless. I sat in sheer and utter dismay. How had all of this happened? Where had everything gone wrong?

Up until this point, I truly thought my husband loved me and wanted to be with me. However, his response was a clear indication that he did not want to remain married to me. After asking if he would be home for the weekend, he replied, "yes". This gave me hope that we could still potentially work through this pitfall in our marriage. He never returned to our home.

As time went on, I made the executive decision that I was going to be happy, and I wasn't going to be with someone who was unhappy. I proceeded with a formal divorce from my husband. After only 18 months of marriage, I could not believe that it had come to this. I was ashamed. I was hurt. My heart was broken into pieces. How was I ever going to recover from this?

How could something that was so good turn into a nightmare in such a short amount of time? Then the whole truth came out.

I discovered that my husband of one year and three months was actually not legally married to his first wife. We were in fact legally married. There was, however, another woman in question. She was a fellow colleague of my husband who had become his mistress. I was being cheated on. This revelation pushed the knife even further in my heart because I had never thought infidelity would have been a problem in my marriage. In fact, my former husband had told me that cheating was the reason he left his first wife. The most disheartening part about this story was that I felt robbed of my time and good intentions. I had fallen in love with a man who didn't genuinely love me in return.

The divorce from my husband and his disappearance prior to the divorce, could have sent me mentally over the edge. A part of me was grateful that I had had the surgery before my relationship exploded. I was an emotional eater; therefore, I'm certain I would have eaten myself way beyond the 400-pound mark.

However, my new stomach wouldn't allow me to emotionally overeat, so I had to tackle this mountain in other ways. I started by digging deep inside myself and aligning my thoughts, actions and beliefs with who I really was. I had to find my identity for certain. I could not let the title of ex-wife define me. I had to rediscover my purpose, and realize that even my divorce was apart of this purpose. It hurt like hell and even got to me mentally. But I had to fight through the battlefield of the mind. I set out to heal the hurts from my childhood, get rid of soul ties and break the cycle of mental, physical, spiritual and financial poverty once and for all.

After my divorce was finalized, I spread my wings and began to fly. I took back my voice from obesity and I took back the life that a lie had stolen from me. The divorce didn't break me. It only made me stronger and helped me to better cultivate my pursuit to live out my purpose. My unexpected divorce could have easily taken me out. I could have been taken under by the trauma and weight of negative emotions. But, I chose life, and the abundance that I knew I had a God-given right to.

My husband's absence pre and post weight loss surgery could not have been worst timing. But surprisingly enough, what I experienced in my marriage was not uncommon. Most bariatric doctors are very candid about surgery and its overall effect on marriages. In fact, losing one's marriage is the number one side effect cited when a spouse undergoes sleeve weight loss. Crazy huh? It is said that an ideal relationship has to be rock solid in order to weather the changes that come along with such a life-altering surgery. Individuals contemplating weight loss surgery within a marriage must engage in in-depth discussions about how the other spouse would honestly feel about their partner losing (or gaining) a significant amount of weight. These conversations can reveal hidden truths that were never summoned to the surface.

If you find yourself in similar situation as the one I experienced, you must remember that your decision to sleeve is one that will dramatically improve your health and livelihood. With that said, sometimes we have to sacrificially separate ourselves from people and circumstances in order to properly care for and save ourselves. Bishop T.D. Jakes once said, "If someone wants to go, let them go." I completely agree with him. Although it may be a hard pill to swallow, your destiny, path and/or journey may not be tied to them.

Veronica's Story

Throughout my sleevin' journey, I have met so many beautiful people with unique stories to share. One of those people is Veronica. With her permission, I would like to take a moment to share her sleevivorship story.

Hello, I'm Veronica, and I am addicted to food. I have fought a journey of obesity for most of my adult life. I was considered "thick" in high school and the first part of college. But then life happened. I lost my grandmother who raised me from 17 months old until I was 21, so I ate to comfort myself. My estranged mother who had come home for my granny's burial tried to seduce my husband, so I ate to combat the pain of betrayal.

My husband left the home my granny left for me to sit in the parking lot of my job in the cold with my baby girl wrapped in a quilt because he didn't want any problems with my mother. She then became verbally abusive towards him after he wouldn't sleep with her; so I ate to help with the anger. Before long, I was using food to comfort myself through any crisis whether it concerned work, home, relationships, children; whatever. Food became my weapon of mass destruction.

As a young African American woman, I was taught to eat whatever was given to me because my family lived below the poverty level. So ham hocks, greens, fat back, macaroni and cheese, chocolate cake, you name it were a regular on the menu in my house. If it had fat, grease, cheese or icing included in the recipe, we ate it. Now back then, my granny would give us castor oil every Friday and we thought it was to keep us healthy from colds or flu type illnesses. Later on, I discovered that this remedy helped flush out all the fatty foods we had consumed during the week as well as potential cold related symptoms.

So how does one change her eating habits to lose weight when she realizes the weight she is carrying is killing her softly? The truth is, I couldn't do it alone and maintain my weight loss. After each heart break or relationship demise, I would start walking, exercising and eating healthier only to lose about 40-50 pounds. I'd regain all the weight back, however, once I got comfortable or fell into another doomed relationship. So eventually I decided to make a permanent change to my life. I started conducting research, and as a nurse, I had witnessed the downside of weight loss surgery. When a gastric bypass had gone bad, some patients were left to endure Total Parenteral Nutrition (TPN), where they receive all their nutrition intravenously *through a feeding tube. And others suffered from open abdominal wounds that never healed and multiple infections. You name it, I saw it. These early experiences led me to put off weight loss surgery. At that point, I was unaware that other methods of bariatric surgery were available. They were not without risk, but these alternatives were not as detrimental as the gastric bypass.*

I continued my research and talking to people. I eventually learned about the gastric sleeve from a good friend of mine. She didn't want anyone to know about her surgery because of the negative stigma associated with it. She didn't want people to criticize her for taking "the easy way out." Even though, there is nothing easy about weight loss surgery! All the counting, measuring, weighing, crying, screaming and laughing to maintain oneself daily is enough to make anyone crazy. But, I eventually followed her lead and underwent gastric sleeve surgery.

I made this decision because it was my way of choosing life. Do I have regrets? Yes, I do, but the benefits far outweigh the regrets. I also wanted my daughters to know that I was willing to do everything humanly possible to live a longer life so I could help raise my grandchildren. Through the emotional and physical domestic violence I suffered, I'm still standing. I want to quit sometimes, but I remember that if God be for me, then who can be against me? In closing, I have a massive and wonderful support system and have led several friends on their weight loss surgery journey. Life is good when we're our healthiest!

Sleevin Ain't Easy Relationship FACTS

- The fact is roughly 50% of all marriages in the US end in divorce.
- The divorce rate is closer to 80% within 2-years for weight loss surgery patients.
- Divorce is considered a side effect of weight loss surgery.

Sleevin Support

As a sleever, you will require four levels of support. I discovered these required areas of support before, during and after my weight loss surgery. Ultimately, strong support in these four areas will determine your ability to remain focused and motivated throughout our journey.

Support Level 1- Mental Support

The battle is won or lost in the mind. Your mentality and thoughts are really ground zero when it comes to support. As you embark upon the re-creation of self and who you know yourself to be before and after weight loss surgery, the integrity of your mental clarity must be maintained. It will be common to wage mental warfare against food, skewed self-perceptions, doubt and even regrets.

When I felt like I wasn't pretty and I verbalized these feelings, I needed support helping me to remember to say and proclaim the opposite. A few weeks after my gastric sleeve surgery, I began gaining weight. This triggered feelings of depression and regret. I just could not figure out what I was doing wrong. I was eating like I was supposed to, taking my vitamins and walking everyday. And I still was gaining weight. It wasn't until I got a personal trainer who recommended that I eat every three hours, that things turned around. I realized, I wasn't eating enough. And as a person who could only eat a few ounces and be satisfied, my body had literally no fuel to burn. This simple paradigm shift and enlightenment about my diet did wonders for my mental clarity.

Support Level 2- Physical Support

Physical support is very important to your success as well after gastric sleeve surgery. In order to see your desired results, it's important to workout and engage in physical activity at least 30 minutes every day. To make this process more successful, acquiring an accountability partner or joining a buddy group will help keep you motivated and encouraged on the days when you don't want to workout. I definitely needed support in this area. I went from being completely inactive to creating a new normal that included regular physical activity. I needed someone to encourage me to keep going on my slow or defiant days. I also needed someone to remind me that I was doing a good job when the accolades were earned. I even needed someone to reprimand me when I did not get up and go to the gym, or was eating something I had no business consuming. I needed a partner to go on this journey with me; needless to say, I had no one but myself. This is why writing this book and starting a community is so important to me. No one should ever have to go on this journey alone like I did.

Support Level 3 - Emotional Support

Emotional support is all about connection and affection. There were times on my journey when I really needed someone to hug me, tell me I was pretty and reassure me that I was doing a great job. I needed to be celebrated every time I lost two, three, four or five pound or achieved a monthly post-surgery milestone.

Having consistent emotional support will help you overcome the disappointment of seeing the number on the scale increase or stay the same. It's important to have individuals around who will be both your cheerleaders and shoulders to cry on. The road to becoming a new you is paved with difficulties, but having a sound emotional support system can help smooth out your path.

Support Level 4-Spiritual Support

Some may forget or negate he spiritual support required to make a lifestyle change. But, let me explain. There is a battle naturally and spiritually that comes with creating a whole new self-reality amid identification. Your flesh, or physical self may want to continue the cycle of emotionally eating when bored or stressed. But, your spirit must be resilient when fighting these desires and temptations. This is why spiritual support is so necessary.

Enlisting a prayer partner to pray with you on the days that are tough and full of regrets is a great way to receive spiritual support. There were days when I felt like I had made the wrong decision and to be spiritually lifted. The motivation and support I needed were far beyond physical, mental or emotional levels. I believe, that there are some forms of emptiness that can only be fulfilled by spiritual renewal from God, and those who help support you on this level.

CHAPTER 5: FINDING MEMO

"To know thyself is the beginning of wisdom".

Socrates

September 27, 2015

Today, I feel really down. Every time I step on the scale, the numbers are increasing instead of decreasing. I don't know what is wrong because I am doing everything right to the "T" of each phase of this new eating lifestyle. I kinda regret even making this decision, because I am not seeing success. My emotions are up and down, because I see all these people who have had this surgery and they are steadily losing and I am gaining. I called Dr. Williams and told him; his nurse said to stay away from the scale and make sure I am drinking my 64 oz of water each day. I can barely drink eight ounces of water in a day let alone 64 oz, which is required of all weight loss surgery patients.

I can't remember when I have ever felt so low. I am generally an upbeat and happy person, but this battle is getting the best of me today. I just have to keep saying everyday that I can do ALL THINGS! My family has been my biggest help, they have been here for me throughout every phase of my obese life, and they are here even more now to see that I win the battle of obesity.

My mama bought me the nastiest calcium vitamins in the world. LOL. But they are all nasty except the very expensive caramel ones that only have fifteen in a pack. Like really though? However, I have to take these things for the rest of my life right along with these multivitamins and B12 supplements. I HATE TAKING PILLS! Ughhh!

I really just want to know my purpose and who I truly am. I don't know who I am. I just know what I am and that is fat and obese. My obesity has defined my mentality towards myself, but I know that there is more to me than food.

Throughout this journey and new lifestyle change, I can say it has taken me on a path that was needed and in the direction of truly finding ME. When you have been a slave to food and obesity for so long, you lose yourself along with your true identity. You are no longer the person that was born with a big imagination and bright ideas when obesity steals everything that you imagined you would be right in front of your very eyes. You'll fight to be unseen and seen at the same time. I know this sounds crazy, but it is true.

There was a little girl back in 1988 whose given name was Miss T. She was pecan brown with long thick pigtails. Miss T. was different from all the other little girls she played with including those in her family. She was overweight so going outside to play any game that required running was not her thing. On one particularly sunny summer afternoon, while at home the phone rang. Not knowing that answering that call would change the trajectory of her whole being Miss T answered. "Hello?" she stated. The voice on the other end was one that she didn't quite recognize. "Hey, is this is the pretty one?" a husky voice asked on the other end. "This is Tib" Miss T answered implying that she wasn't the pretty one. The caller responded, "I know who this is. You are the pretty one," he laughed. "Is your daddy at home? This is Mr. Jerry Wright. Can you get him to the phone? Miss T walked to the door and yelled out to her daddy that Mr. Jerry was on the phone for him. With the biggest smile on her face she returned to the line to let him know that her dad was on his way.

If you hadn't figured it out, Miss T is me, and that is a day that I will never forget. It was the first time I had ever had a male figure tell me that I was pretty. I didn't think of myself as pretty because I was fat. Being fat shamed constantly created a blanket of self-hate that I wore around daily. But memories like these helped me to realize the beauty that I overlooked even when others saw it shining through.

Mirror Mirror

As I mentioned in a previous chapter, I had to undergo a psych evaluation before my weight loss surgery. This was to make sure that I was not only mentally strong for weight loss surgery, but life after as well. Your mind and what you see in the mirror will have to adjust as your body changes. Accordingly, I live by the following quote:

"Discovering who you are is only the beginning,

functioning in who you are will align you to your purpose to fulfill your destiny." Tiberia Morris

To move in greatness and discover who you really are means to purposely maintain and operate in an emotional, mental and spiritual state that is conducive to establishing influence and affluence in the world. Your level of greatness depends on knowing who you are and that greatness is inside you no matter what size you are. Whatever you believe is possible in your life is yours to have and that includes overcoming obesity.

As you grow in faith and move in sync with who you are becoming along your weight loss journey, there are steps you can take that will help fully maximize your strides. These actions will determine whether your sown seeds of consistency and discipline will return 30, 60 or 100 times on your efforts. My personal journey took me to a place I had not wanted to go, and that was within.

Many times we fail to look inward and examine whether or not our inner world is unbalanced. Like any journey it requires one to examine their mental house. Winning against obesity is all about the battle of the mind. In fact, I truly believe that our minds in conjunction with our actions can either create a life of wins or losses. Once I became truthful with myself and about what I had done to my body, then I was able to go inward and deal with the self hate and increase my level of self love towards who I was becoming.

I had to love all of me internally in order to fully love my external self. I had to view myself through the eyes of God to realize that I was a priceless treasure. And you have to do the same. No longer settle for what your mind may be negatively telling you about your results or stage in your journey. Your mind is a powerful tool that was designed to push you beyond that which has been previously planted. That means negative vibes, energies and people can be overcome. I knew success in the mental realm was my first order of business if I ever were to meet the girl I had always longed know and experience life as.

9 Daily Tips To Overcome Obesity And Discover Who You Are

Tip 1: Evolution is Key

You must evolve. Evolving will require your committed willingness to change. According to the dictionary, evolve means to develop gradually, especially from a simple to a more complex form. There is nothing simple or ordinary about a person with greatness. You must be willing to unlearn everything that you were taught about you if it is not conducive to your evolution. This will take great courage and strength because you will have to unmask all of your insecurities and become vulnerable with yourself.

I have adopted a saying to help with my personal evolution process. Truth answers ALL THINGS. We must be honest with ourselves when understanding and learning who we really are. Remembering that God is the Master of creation and evolution will aid us in this process. His word causes us to grow and evolve when we stand on its truth. And when we believe in the word of God, we literally become new creations, dying to our former selves. Learn what the word says about you, accept it and walk out its mandates. This is the sacred course of spiritual evolution.

Tip 2: Celebrate A Birth And Funeral

In order to discover who you really are you must be willing to bury the old you in order to resurrect the new you. Sounds very similar to what Jesus did when he died on the cross for our sins in order that we may be resurrected as new creatures in him. I know this may sound like an odd task, but I had to engage and celebrate both a funeral and rebirth in every area of my life. Literally, no area was off limits.

Tip 3: Anticipate Victory

Remember that at the end of every trial is a triumph! Discovering who you are will not always be peaches and cream. Therefore, be patient with yourself. While maneuvering through your journey to beat obesity, there will be times that you may stop exercising or even eat the wrong kinds of food. Don't beat yourself up about it. If you can remember that you are a person on a journey with ups and downs who will eventually experience success, you have what it takes to weather any storm.

Tip 4: Be Extremely Honest

Be honest with YOU! Oftentimes, we are not totally honest with ourselves concerning our personalities, thoughts, needs, wants and desires. As you discover your true self, honesty is key. I had to admit that I didn't know myself, and that for much of my life I had allowed obesity to be my identity. Fat was my only definition of self. It wasn't until I was honest about this fact that I could finally get to know who I truly was outside of the obesity storyline I had hid behind.

Tip 5: Never Confuse Obesity With A Curse Or Laziness

Obesity is not a curse meant to keep you from living life. For many years, I thought that being fat was a punishment and just the way I was destined to live. I couldn't see my life beyond my "fat suit". Oftentimes, the greatest version of ourselves is covered up by the physical, emotional and mental manifestations that we are meant to conquer. Obesity is one of them.

Just because you are overweight doesn't mean you are lazy. Nor does it mean that choosing to have weight loss surgery is a lazy cop out. you should never view yourself other than anyone who embodies greatness and the necessary tools for success. Challenges are inevitable, but their presence in our lives should never make us feel like we're lazy or cursed. You are always capable at succeeding at whatever you believe is possible.

Tip 6: Ask Questions

Question everything, especially on the topic of you. Don't limit the depth or height of your questioning either. Push beyond what you have always done in the hopes of accomplishing something new in life. Stepping outside your box and comfort zone will open up possibilities you never knew existed. Don't be afraid to seek out a completely new vision of self.

Tip 7: Trust God

When embarking on your journey of self discovery, trust God. More importantly, trust the God in you. Know that you will not fail. This is such a simple concept, but sometimes we trust everything beyond and instead of the spirit of God that resides within us. We trust that if we go to work from 9 to 5 every day, we will receive a check at the end of the week. We never give thought that something could go wrong with payroll. Then why can't we trust the God in us in the same manner when it comes to our lives?

Tip 8: Get Balanced

Learning and maintaining mental and spiritual equilibrium is a game changer! It's important to know that you are a spiritual being having a human experience. This outlook is known as the God perspective on life. When you view yourself, circumstances and battle with obesity from God's viewpoint, it is easier to strategize and succeed over your enemy.

Tip 9: Recognize The Origin Of Greatness

Greatness comes from the core of who you are. Once you identify who you are, then you can identify your greatness. I have been extremely blessed to have a number of people enter and exit my life. They all played a role in determining the trajectory of who I am and the Tiberia I am becoming.

CHAPTER 6: WINNING WITHIN

Undergoing a major weight loss surgery brought about life-altering changes. I went through physical, emotional and spiritual states of being that I had never before experienced. The changes in my body uncovered emotions about myself, life, relationships and goals that were foreign to me. I had been so consumed by obesity for so much of my life that I had never really considered ever fighting and winning over the battle of the bulge. For this reason, I had to learn to develop a winning mindset. This change in my thinking patterns is what kept me on course emotionally and mentally when I didn't see instant results after my surgery. However, having a winning mindset helped me to not only trust, but love the process of my weight loss journey.

There is a distinct life that I had before my gastric sleeve surgery and the one I experience now post-operation. The mindset that I had about food, life, goals and challenges has now been replaced with new thoughts about these subjects. I've learned that having weight loss surgery required me to create a victory-based storyline within myself. This process of turning negative, self-deprecating thoughts into ones that nourish my soul was not an easy task. It was a daily assignment that I had to tackle like my life depended on it. Because in all actuality, my livelihood was indeed on the line.

Societally speaking, many of us disregard the importance of celebrating ourselves. We are taught that such an act is boastful, arrogant or the exact opposite of godly humility. But, I learned that celebrating both my small and large victories helped me to progress successfully in my life after weight loss surgery. Finding joy in personal victories refreshes the soul and gives us the energy we need to troubleshoot the obstacles and hardships that may come our way. Without instilling the practice of celebrating our wins, we easily miss out on the everlasting joy that God promised all of his children here on earth and forevermore. Lauryn Hill said it best in her song Doo Wop: "How you gon' win if you ain't right within?"

It is each and everyone of our personal responsibility to create an internally-sound winning mindset. This victorious way of thinking will lead to the success stories that we all desire. So whether it's undergoing weight loss surgery, writing a book, starting a business or meeting the love of our lives, the journey always begins with a positive mindset and outlook on life. When you have set your mental compass towards victory, you will more clearly discern the direction that is most beneficial for your life's mission.

Before I had focused my mindset on victory, I had created a world that was the root cause of my obesity. As a child, I had never imagined being so overweight that it would become hard for me to physically walk or rest well at night. And even when I was put on a CPAP machine to help me breathe at night, my negatively-focused mindset blinded me from seeing the potential that I am now experiencing in life. I now realize that building a winning mindset, first requires us to unearth the traumas that we have buried deep in the back of our minds. For me, coming to grips with the pain of being touched inappropriately by a relative as a child was probably one of the hardest emotional and mental tasks of my life. But, bringing light to this trauma helped me uncover other emotional traumas that had ultimately led to my physical weight gain. Issues like the absenteeism of my biological father, or my overwhelming desire to be wanted and loved by the opposite sex, and my growing obsession and adoration for food over individuals or mutually beneficial relationships all came bubbling to the surface. And when they were brought to light, I finally gave myself the opportunity to confront, deal with and heal from their wounds.

We all, at one time or another, have experienced the enemy within ourselves. Sometimes we allow doubts, hopelessness and negative self-talk to utterly consume us. However, we can only overcome this internal battle when we challenge its standards. Sometimes this means confronting the thoughts, beliefs and circumstances that we were taught to believe as normal by people who raised and love us. For me, this meant challenging how my grandmother used food as her love language. She was sincere in her desire to feed her family, but my personal struggle of replacing actual love with food was a stronghold that I had to eradicate. When I did, I knew it was my mission to share the ramifications of this journey with others.

CHAPTER 7: PURPOSELY EMERGED

The sleeved life was one I was anxiously excited about, yet I knew it was going to be challenging to free myself from what had been my hell on earth experience. I discovered, while adapting to the sleeved life, that even as my body was changing and adjusting to the results of my surgery, my mind had to catch up with it. For example, I never really knew that eating and drinking at the same time would be a task that I would have to give up. The day I learned that I would no longer be able to do the two simultaneously, I began to question everything. In America, we have grown so accustomed to washing down our food with an icy cold beverage. Our minds are trained to see food and drink as a packaged deal. But after my surgery, I realized that having a beverage with every meal was a freedom that I would have to give up. Nowadays, I actually don't even drink anything most times after a meal.

Beyond changing my eating routine, I was formally introduced to a version of myself that I had never met before. It was almost like being a new baby who had to learn to walk and talk again. There were so many hidden things about myself that obesity had buried alive. And just like a butterfly breaking from its cocoon after discovering it has wings, I began to fly! Adapting to a smaller body was emotional for me at first. Because even though I was 135 pounds lighter, I still at times felt like the 385-pound woman when I looked in the mirror. This mental body dysmorphia, would then result in self-neglect and abuse. This was a cycle that I had to break early on because the woman I always longed to be had to kill the woman I had grown accustomed to being. It was during these battles in my mirror, however, that I finally identified my purpose.

For years, I had always viewed my obesity as a curse. It wasn't until I took the steps to beat obesity, that I realized this struggle was actually a part of my divine purpose and path. I know it might sound crazy, but I really believe that my battle with obesity was designed for me to conquer. As a result, I can now help countless others in the world who are eating to live and fighting to lose just like me.

In order for my purpose to emerge from the fats of life, I had to do five things.

1. Admit that I had an eating addiction
2. Identify the triggers of the eating addiction
3. Kick fear in the butt
4. Decide to do what I felt right in my heart/spirit concerning my health
5. Wait No More

The fact that my purpose had been inside of me all along makes me sad for former versions of Tiberia. She had allowed how she physically looked on the outside to keep her from seeing the truth of her personal beauty and life's work. I now have the tools to make sure I never again endure such a misappropriation of my God-given purpose. Now that I know my purpose is to speak out about obesity and surgery shaming, I have changed how I view obesity as a whole. Obesity isn't a life sentence. And at any given moment, anyone battling obesity can bail his or herself out without the help of a bondsman.

I was only able to get into this space by creating a routine of being alone with myself. This "Me Time" helped me to fully heal. During this quiet time I realized that I was not only recovering from surgery and my emerging new body. I was also getting over the trauma of my divorce. I really had to evaluate how I was utilizing my 24 hours each day. Where I was spending my time and who I was spending it with became very important to me. Getting clarity in the area of time management helped me realize that many of us miss out on intimately getting acquainted with ourselves because we spend little to no time with ourselves. I came to realize that there was no difference between the time I have in a day and that which is used by Oprah. How she prioritizes her time is the only difference. Essentially, we can no longer waste time on things that do not concern our purpose.

We must budget time specifically to spend in our own sacred presence. Doing this allowed me to better articulate my core values, and what I need and want in platonic and romantic relationships. Spending the necessary time with yourself allows total healing to take place. I knew that from my years of the war with obesity there were some areas in my life that had gone undealt with for many years. I encourage you to take as much time as you need in your own presence so that you can heal from any tragedies that may have been a deriving factor of the imprisonment of obesity.

Finding who I am has been one of my greatest rewards. This journey wasn't easy because I was hidden behind a fat suit that I had sewn for myself. In spite of this however, obesity became the pattern that God used to knit me together; this was all my creation. Every day I lived a life submerged under pain, hurts, rejection, abuse and negative thoughts. I was drowning and didn't even realize that I was the one holding myself down. I was committing the suicide of my purpose and destiny.

Just imagine yourself being held under water. You're

flailing and gasping for air. The only way you can come up is if you allow yourself to. This is what some of you are doing to your purpose when you refuse to emerge from the pain of your past, childhood hurts, rejection and negative self talk. Decide now to let yourself emerge and breathe again.

CHAPTER 8: WHAT ABOUT YOUR FRIENDS?

One would think that having a circle of friends would mean that we'd all have a built-in support system of cheerleaders, fans and encouragers. Especially after undergoing something as life-altering as weight loss surgery. But what happens when your friends don't live up to any of those expectations? The 90s girl group, TLC, had it right with their hit song, What About Your Friends? What I learned, and want to share is that as a sleevivor sister you will lose friends. Now, I can't say that this applies to sleevivor brothers too, because I don't think men get jealous of their male friends after massive weight loss.

I was always the biggest girl in my circle of friends and we always supported one another. My group even cheered me on when I made the decision to undergo weight loss surgery and are still my companions now. However, there have been several cases where people have lost truly close friends after having gastric sleeve surgery and losing astronomical amounts of weight. In fact, I have met countless sleevivors who share the heartbreaking story of losing friends after weight loss. And people wonder why many bariatric patients hide our decision to undergo surgery in the first place. Surgery shaming is real. Hence, many people have chosen to get sleeved in secrecy, thus having no close support system during or after their procedure.

So what is the reason for this? Most sleevivors have said they were always the overweight girl within their sister circle or circle of friends. Their friends had grown accustomed to the sleevivor being the "fat one"; until she decided that she didn't want to live that type of lifestyle anymore. Not telling your friends your decision to undergo weight loss surgery because of the fear of being talked out of it or not positively is difficult. This is a BIG STEP and decision to make alone. As mentioned in previous chapters, a support system helps tremendously and is needed. I found it so disheartening as I scrolled social media to read the stories of fellow sleevivors whose supposedly good and solid friendships of many years had gone up in flames all because they chose to save their lives and get healthy.

I can't say that I have personally experienced losing friends because of weight loss surgery, but I have lost friends and I know how much losing this type of relationship hurts. It's painful to know that a person you were once in close relationship with decides to sever ties with you because they feel that you've chosen a new identity over their friendship. Life changing moments like surgery, will really show you the truth about individuals in your circle. However, I want to encourage you if you have lost friends on your new life transformation journey that there are a host of beautiful, friendly and great sleevivor sisters in the world who will give you all the support you need. I am one of them.

My ultimate goal is to build and fortify the sleevivor sisterhood in every state. Having a band of women who celebrate and not just tolerate your decision to undergo weight loss surgery and live a new life is imperative. I want to see that you reach every daily, weekly, monthly and yearly goal that you have set for yourself. And when you make your happiness and health your top priority, I can promise you that the right friends and partners will enter your life.

There will be highs and lows in this sleeved life. I truly believe if we conquered the fear of doing this surgery, we can definitely conquer anything else we desire to defeat. In the next few pages I will share a story of a woman who has had the gastric sleeve and how things changed with not just friends, but family as well.

BE CAREFUL WHO YOU TELL ABOUT YOUR WEIGHT LOSS SURGERY

This story is from Lisa of California.

I just had gastric sleeve surgery three weeks ago. I have to say, the first week out I realized that my life had truly changed. I don't cook as much for my family anymore because I'm not hungry as much, or am restricted to a liquid diet. Therefore, the common happenings of cooking and smelling food in the house is not as frequent, which I think my son misses. Cooking was a relaxing part of my life; I miss it too.

I have now started cooking homemade meals again because my family needs to eat. The problem I have had is with my mother. The surgery has become a point of contention between her and I. I feel so alone on this journey and I'm trying to navigate my way with my new stomach and eating habits. My mother has been very critical. She does not understand the surgery, even though she is a medical professional. She constantly badgers me about what I consume and drink. I tell her that I cannot drink a whole cupful of soup in one sitting. With this surgery you have to take small baby sips of liquid, as I told her my stomach can only hold about 1 - 2 ounces. She goes ballistic talking about that this is not healthy. "Oh, my God" as she states, followed by the ongoing criticism about the surgery.

When I was dieting on my own, my mother would always ask "What are you doing about the weight?" Now that I have done something, she is not supportive and can't and will never understand my decision because she weighs 150 pounds. So, overall, I have had to keep this to myself. I will only communicate with people who have had the surgery or are about to go on this journey. I will not tell anyone else in my family or friends other than the three people I already told.

I think if I tell a lot of people there will be unsolicited accountability interjected into my life. People will expect me to be slim extremely quick because I had surgery. But what happens if I don't lose all the weight? I think I need to be accountable to myself for weight loss and not other people. It should be understood that some people will never try to understand what their loved one is going through before and after weight loss surgery. So I say be careful about who you share your weight loss decisions with.

CHAPTER 9: FLIGHT 1430

How long will you wait to lose the extra weight? How long will you wait to change the life that you created for yourself to the one you truly desire? How long will you wait to live your abundance now life? The one thing I regret most about having weight loss surgery is not doing it soon enough. I waited and pushed it off all because of the fear of not waking from the anesthesia, or failing yet another attempt to lose weight.

There is indeed an art to waiting, and it is even necessary in some situations. However, waiting has been one of the major killers of people's goals, dreams, desires and needs. Waiting is merely a classy word that is dating procrastination. You may be saying, "I've got to wait until my finances are together before I can launch my business." You may even be saying, "I have to wait until I lose some weight before I can launch my speaking career." I said all of these things and they were just excuses that I chose to use to hide my fears of why I really didn't want to do the surgery. I watched others from afar who took their life back and said they will not wait anymore on doing something that will enhance and create the life they wanted. I was inspired by their stories. They gave me the push I needed to take my final leap of faith.

Wait No More is more than just a mere phrase written in a book. This is a movement I will be launching across the country and social media worlds. *Wait No More* isn't about weight loss, it is about the four major core elements of life. This movement address the four areas of life where we all need to put aside waiting and get moving.

These areas are
1. Physically
2. Mentally
3. Spiritually
4. Financially

Why wait any longer in any of those areas of your life? Waiting is the thief to the manifestation of a life being lived on top of a hill. Time is one thing we all have been given, but how much time we don't know. So why waste it waiting!

I kept putting my decision off to have gastric sleeve surgery, and my hoping and praying wasn't working. I had to do something. I was waiting on God, but He was waiting on me to stop being afraid and move. Oftentimes, we put off what can be accomplished today as an assignment for tomorrow. But for many of us, tomorrow never comes because we procrastinate. Before we know it, years have passed and we are still in the same spot or position we have been in for years.

How long will you continue to put yourself on the back burner and neglect to live the life you want to live in good health? Yes, it is easier said than done, but nothing comes without a challenge or work. Wait no more on living the life you desire. Don't allow another day to go by without doing one thing to produce the change you want to see in your physical, financial, spiritual, mental or emotional worlds. Decide to say I do to your greatness and destiny today. The woman or man inside of you is longing to come forth. Allow them to emerge so that you can help others emerge too.

CHAPTER 10: WAIT NO MORE

One of my greatest victories on my journey was taking my first trip on an airplane. To some this may seem trivial or small, but for me this was a defining moment in my life. I had always wanted to fly somewhere; it didn't matter where, I just wanted to fly. I know you probably are thinking well just buy the ticket and go. I wished it was that simple, but living as an obese person things this small weren't so simple. My fear wasn't of flying per se. I was actually more afraid of flying fat and having to purchase two seats or not being able to put on the seat belt. I had heard stories of people who were either unable to fly or had to pay double for a seat because of their morbid obesity.

April 10, 2016 will be a day I will never forget. I weighed the lightest I had ever been in my adult life at 253 pounds. I could cross my legs and was wearing a size 18 in clothing. Sitting at my dining room table, booking my first flight was such a surreal moment. Never did I imagine that I would be getting ready to take my first flight. Experiencing the very thing I had always longed for was a very overwhelming feeling. It literally felt like the night before Christmas when I was about to leave for my trip. I couldn't sleep a wink. I was like a kid waiting on Santa Claus to arrive. The ride to the airport the next day was a thrill in itself. Arriving to the departure drop off location made my dreams become real. I, Tiberia Sheree Morris, was about to navigate her way through the Atlanta Hartsfield Airport by herself and get on a plane.

I know this may sound so minute to you, but for an obese person this was huge. Yes, I could have flown long before I did. Losing weight is not a prerequisite to flying. However, when you are obese the mental and emotional battle that ensues can be overwhelming and downright petrifying.

That day I experienced one of my greatest victories. I fit into an airplane seat comfortably and was able to fasten my seat belt without needing an extender. Not to mention, I could cross my legs too! YASSSSS, to the crossing of the legs! Between that and being able to wear leggings in public, honey I was straight slaying. This was pure V-I-C-T-O-R-Y!

ABOUT THE AUTHOR

Tiberia Morris is a minister and motivational speaker who resides in the beautiful city of Atlanta by way of Rome, Georgia. As the founder of EmergHer, Morris endeavors to help women emerge from mediocrity into the fullness of self, mentally, physically, spiritually and financially. To learn more about Tiberia Morris and her personal and professional missions for life, visit www.tiberiamorris.com.

www.ingramcontent.com/pod-product-compliance
Lightning Source LLC
Chambersburg PA
CBHW061710250726
48657CB00002B/579